Antibiotic and Antiviral Ingredients and Recipes

A Guide to Treating Infections Naturally

Disclaimer and Terms of Use:

Effort has been made to ensure that the information in this book is accurate and complete, however, the author and the publisher do not warrant the accuracy of the information, text and graphics contained within the book due to the rapidly changing nature of science, research, known and unknown facts and internet. The Author and the publisher do not hold any responsibility for errors, omissions or contrary interpretation of the subject matter herein. This book is presented solely for motivational and informational purposes only.

Table of Contents

Introduction

I want to thank you and congratulate you for downloading the book, *"Antibiotic and Antiviral Ingredients and Recipes: A Guide to Treating Infections Naturally"*.

We have been relying on antibiotic and antiviral medications to treat various infections ever since these miracle drugs became commercially available. While they do indeed seem to work miracles when it comes to providing relief for common illnesses, the way they affect our body in the long run may not be so worth it. The good thing is Mother Nature herself has already given us what we need if we are looking for relief.

This book first explains how antibiotics and antiviral medications work and then moves on to suggest why going for natural ingredients is the better option for treatment. It then lists down a number of natural antibiotic and antiviral ingredients that are mostly found in your kitchen cabinets. Finally, you will learn about some recipes that are not only delicious, but are also effective in getting rid of infections and treating common illnesses.

Thanks again for downloading this book, I hope you enjoy it!

Chapter 1 | How Antibiotics and Antiviral Medications Work

People didn't have a lot of options for treating infections before laboratory made antibiotics and antiviral medications came about. Today, antibiotics are widely used against bacterial infections such as strep throat, pneumonia, or bacterial bronchitis. Antiviral medications, on the other hand, are used to ward off viral infections such as the common cold, influenza or gastroenteritis.

The advancing state of technology has now allowed us to discover and create more of these kinds of drugs, thus giving us more ways to keep ourselves protected from various diseases. Before people had access to these, however, they made use of natural ingredients that had antibiotic and antiviral properties.

Antibiotics and Antiviral Medications

Friendly bacteria live inside the human body, and they make sure that nothing goes wrong with our digestive system. Aside from that, they also regulate metabolism and keep the immune system working at its best. However, there will be moments when their vicious relatives attack our systems and cause infections that may sometimes even be life threatening. Oftentimes, our doctors prescribe antibiotic medications to treat diseases caused by these bad bacteria. The type of bacterial infection will determine which antibiotic will be prescribed to us.

Antibiotics usually kill off bacteria in three ways: 1) by blocking the bacteria's ability to build a cell wall; 2) by preventing the bacteria's ribosomes from building new proteins; and 3) by inhibiting the bacteria from repairing its broken DNA strands. Most antibiotics available in the market today are what we call "broad spectrum", or those that can fight off various kinds of bacteria.

On the other hand, those that target specific kinds of bacteria are called "narrow spectrum" antibiotics. When these medications are taken in, they enter the bloodstream and move through the body to kill bacteria, making sure that they are not harming human cells. However, the problem with this is that even the good bacteria are wiped out in the process. More of this disadvantage will be discussed in the following chapter.

Viruses, on the other hand, differ from bacteria in that they are not comprised of any cells. Instead, they are made up of DNA or RNA strands that are enclosed in an envelope of protein known as the capsid. Some of them will even have protective fat layering covering the capsid. Viral infections happen when the virus infiltrates healthy body cells and injects its genetic information into the nucleus. It then uses the cell to make copies of itself, leaving it to infect other healthy cells so that the body gets infected.

Unlike antibiotics, antiviral medications do not kill off the virus, but instead, they work by limiting the virus' capacity to reproduce. This works in two ways. The antiviral blocks the virus from entering the host cell, thus keeping the virus from inserting its genetic material to the healthy cell's nucleus, or they interfere with how the virus spreads from infected cells. When the virus becomes unable to infect your other cells, they tend to lessen and as a result, you feel better because your systems would not have to work extra hard to contain the virus.

When we get sick, perhaps the first kinds of treatment that come to mind are antibiotics or antiviral drugs. After all, these are what the doctors commonly prescribe and true enough, to a large extent, they accomplish the job. Some people may believe that such drugs are the only things that can do the trick, but it is worth knowing that the most common infections can be treated or prevented by ingredients that can be found in the kitchen. In the next chapter, we will discuss the benefits of going for natural antibiotics and antivirals, as well as the ingredients that you can use to make them.

Chapter 2 | The Benefits of Going Natural

Antibiotic and antiviral medications are indeed effective for treating infections. However, they may not be the best options that are available for us today. One of the main reasons why these treatment medications are not as ideal as we think is because of the possible side effects that they can bring. Like most forms of medication, both antibiotic and antiviral medications can cause side effects including, but not limited, to nausea and vomiting, dizziness and even allergic reactions.

When a doctor prescribes you to take in any medication, always ask about the possible side effects that the medicines can result to. In cases where these side effects are experienced, consult your doctor as well if you should or should not continue with the medication. With allergic reactions, for example, it is best to stop the medication and have the doctor prescribe you an alternative right away.

Why Go Natural?

Antibiotics are highly potent and effective in treating bacterial infections. Unfortunately, aside from the possibility of side effects, there are other concerns that you need to consider along with these medications. For one, antibiotics are effective in killing bacteria, but they are too effective in that they also destroy the good bacteria that the body needs. These good and naturally occurring bacteria, when destroyed by antibiotics, are then more prone to be replaced by disease-causing bacteria.

Good bacteria or probiotics as they are called have important functions within the body. One of these is to help with the digestive process, and another is to help fight off the bad bacteria that can cause sickness and diseases. Another reason why it is not advisable to take in antibiotics at the first sign of bacterial infection symptoms is the danger of antibiotic resistance. Antibiotic resistance refers to the building of resistance of disease-causing microbes to antibiotic drugs due to continuous use.

In other words, the more you use antibiotic drugs, the more resistant the bacteria can become towards the medication. Highly resistant bacteria are more difficult to destroy and require even more powerful antibiotics. Of course, more potent antibiotics come at a higher price, but the real danger is in having bacteria that can no longer be treated by the antibiotics that are available to us today.

Suffice to say, antibiotic-resistant bacteria are harder to treat and are more complicated in many ways. Antibiotic-resistant bacteria are able to spread faster and can threaten entire communities with a new kind of infection. These infections also do not respond to regular doses of drugs, making the treatment process more complicated and expensive. Finally, antibiotic resistance can lead ultimately to death as the underlying infections are left untreated.

Side effects, the destruction of good bacteria, and antibiotic resistance are reasons enough to make people think that there should be a better alternative to antibiotic medicines. The good thing is there is. Mother Nature has come up with naturally effective and safe treatments that you can use against bacterial infections, and they have been used for many centuries in traditional medicine.

In the same way that antibiotics can be found in natural and organic materials, there are many herbs and other items that can be found in nature that are effective as antiviral solutions. Most antibiotic agents are also effective against viral infections, making it easier to avoid both kinds of infection with the same types of food. The use of antibiotics has taught us that these drugs are not always the best options for treating infections. On top of avoiding their side effects, there are also other reasons why going the natural path may be the better option.

Viral infections are often manifested by fevers and other common symptoms that make it hard to pinpoint the exact problem. People who show symptoms often have to undergo specific tests to find out what disease they have, losing valuable time and resources.

On an alternate route, those who choose to go for natural antiviral treatments will find it convenient to know that most of these natural remedies are able to act on a large number, if not all types of viral infection. This means that taking one natural treatment could save you from your viral infection, whether it is diarrhea, the common colds, or a form or another of flu.

Additionally, because of the broad spectrum that natural antiviral remedies are able to cover, there are even infections that are very difficult to treat with medications that can be treated much easily with natural antivirals. Some diseases caused by viral infections may not even be treatable with drugs and other pharmaceuticals, but studies have found that there are natural remedies that could actually work on the untreatable diseases.

Another reason why natural antivirals are a better choice is the fact that they are simply convenient. These are natural remedies, meaning they are easily and readily available through local resources. Most antibiotics and antivirals are even part of the normal pantry so all you have to do is reach into your home cabinets. In terms of cost and convenience, natural alternatives are at an advantage over drugs and other pharmaceuticals. Moreover, natural antivirals and antibiotics, even in their capsulated forms, normally have longer shelf lives that make them more effective in the long run.

Natural Antibiotic Ingredients

<u>Garlic</u>

Garlic has a long-standing history of being a great treatment for fungal, bacterial, parasitic and viral infections. During World War II, it was used as a natural and organic remedy against infections. This is because of garlic's active compound, allicin, which has effects very similar to that of penicillin. The natural spice of garlic has strong antibacterial effects, making it effective even against drug-resistant microbes.

To enjoy the antibiotic benefits of garlic, it should be crushed well, left exposed to the air for a couple of minutes, and then eaten raw.

<u>Turmeric</u>

Turmeric is known for its use in the culinary industry, and it has also been found to have outstanding anti-inflammatory and antibacterial effects. This potent spice is also known for its anti-infective and anti-carcinogenic effects, making it a great natural alternative to antibiotic medicines. It is advisable for a person to consume at least 1 to 2 teaspoons of turmeric a day, mixed in to the day's recipes.

<u>Oregano Oil</u>

Oregano oil is marketed as an effective agent against infections and bacteria. Its medicinal purposes include treatment against viral, fungal and bacterial infections, and it is known for effectively strengthening the immune system. To use oregano oil, simply apply 2-3 drops to the infection, about 3-4 times a day. If taken orally in the form of capsules, then 100-150 mg doses are recommended. Some of the cases it has been known to be effective against are acne, diarrhea, colds, athlete's foot and sinusitis.

<u>Olive Leaf</u>

Olive leaves are another natural remedy for bacterial, viral and fungal infections. The active component oleuropein has been found to have therapeutic effects, and it has been used for analgesic purposes. Olive leaves and their extract capsules are also low in toxicity, making them safe to consume on a daily basis. A dosage of 25 mg two times a day is recommended for health maintenance, while an intake of olive leaf extracts three times a day is recommended for the treatment of colds, flu, herpes, sinusitis and allergies.

Tea Tree Oil

Tea tree oil has long been used in traditional medicine as a treatment for skin infections such as acne, scabies, burns and insect bites. As it gets absorbed deeper into the skin, its effects have also been found effective against fungal and bacterial infections. Simply apply the oil to the infected area and leave on to let it sink into the skin. Keep in mind that tea tree oil is for external use only.

Pau d' Arco

Pau d' Arco is a natural herb form South America that is becoming known for its effects against infections. Its active ingredient lapachol is able to bring relief to viral, fungal and bacterial infections. Recent studies have also shown that pau d' arco may have anti-cancer properties, although further investigation is needed. Pau d' arco is a powerful herbal antibiotic that is being used to fight life-threatening diseases. As a maintenance supplement, it is also able to strengthen the immune system, further protecting the body from infections. Pau d' arco is mostly taken in the form of tea by letting the leaves steep in hot water.

Ginger

Ginger is another natural wonder that is oftentimes underappreciated. This culinary ingredient offers a distinct flavor in a wide variety of recipes, and it has been found to have antibacterial effects. Ginger consists of gingerols, shogaol, and zingerone that are known to fight off bacteria. In addition to this, ginger has also long been used in the Ayurvedic medicinal system as it is an effective anti-inflammatory agent, as well as a therapeutic food. Cook food with at least 2-3 inches of ginger for daily maintenance. In the case of bacterial infections, you can take ginger in the form of a hot tea drink by letting a small piece steep in hot water.

Cinnamon and Honey

A combination of cinnamon and honey is a wonderful natural treatment for bacterial infections and diseases. Mix a tablespoon of honey and a teaspoon of cinnamon into your drink and enjoy it hot or cold. This will strengthen the immune system and will help protect the body from viruses and bacteria by fortifying the body's white blood cells. To make sure that you get the full benefits, make sure to use unpasteurized honey as the pasteurization process can destroy some of its active medicinal components.

Vitamin C

    Vitamin C is a known nutrient that can help fight off infections and diseases. Like most vitamins and minerals, vitamin C is naturally available in almost all fresh fruits, especially those from the citrus family. Consumed from this natural state, there is no limit as to how much vitamin C your body can take in. In supplement form, 1-3 grams of daily dosage is recommended. However, in the case of a viral or bacterial issue, increasing the intake of vitamin C is highly recommended.

Natural Antiviral Ingredients

Ginger Root Tea

Ginger root is not only a natural antibiotic, but is an antiviral as well. The herbal extract is used as a remedy for many conditions, with its uses known specifically for respiratory illnesses and as an expectorant. Use ginger root tea to treat allergic rhinitis, allergies, and sinus infections by steeping some chopped ginger in hot water.

Astralagus Extract

Astralagus is an herb that has special beneficial effects on the body's immune system. It increases the body's resistance against infection from virus and bacteria by increasing the count of white blood cells and stimulating the growth of antibodies. Long known for these benefits, this natural remedy is recognized as an immune system herb that has been used in Chinese medicine for the last two thousand years. The herb is still used in many areas as protection before the winter flu season, as well as the spring flu season as well.

Olive Leaf

Olive leaf is one of the most widely effective natural antibiotic and antiviral herbs available. The active component oleuropein hampers the growth of viruses and bacteria, and it actively stimulates the immune system to provide protection against foreign bodies. One special attribute of the olive leaf and its extracts is its capacity to fight off any type of herpes, as well as a list of viral diseases that are deemed untreatable by pharmaceutical drugs such as polio, the coaxsackie virus, and the herpes virus, Epstein barr.

Essential Oils

History proves the effectiveness of essential oils against infectious diseases. Through years and histories, these oils have been used against plagues and pandemics, some of them saving vast communities from the nastiest plagues of all time. Even in nature, oils act as natural agents that protect plants from bacteria, viruses and other harmful microbes. The oils' evolving nature also makes it possible to fight off viruses and bacteria, no matter how they evolve. Some of the essential oils that are in use today are:

1. *Eucalyptus radiata* – A potent antiviral that supports the immune system. It is effective against colds, flu, pneumonia and other infections of the respiratory system.

2. Lemon balm – Scientifically known as *Melissa officinalis*, lemon balm has been scientifically proven as one of the most effective antiviral oils. More than strengthening the immune system, it also proves as a hindrance against viral replication. Lemon balm is effective against throat infections, cold sores and dysentery.

3. Melaleuca Essential Oil – This essential oil is one of the most effective anti-everything oils available today. It is known as an antiviral, antibacterial, antifungal, anti-infectious, and anti-parasitic essential oil. Moreover, it aids in tissue regeneration that helps improve the body's immune system. Those with sensitive skin may find that they need to dilute this oil first, and homeowners might be glad to know that they are good household cleaners, too.

Chapter 3 | Antibiotic Recipes

Bacterial infections are something you have to deal with from time to time, and the time it takes for you to get past them will ultimately be determined by what you eat and how your immune system responds to it. As we already know the bad side effects of relying too much on antibiotic drugs, here are some natural antibiotic recipes that can help you get through those infections in an affordable and completely safe way.

Some of these recipes may not appeal at all to your taste. However, it should be noted that their purpose is not for taste, but for effective relief against diseases.

Antibiotic Tonic

This recipe is a tried and tested formula that keeps bacterial infections at bay and knocks them out as soon as possible. It is recommended to have a masticating juicer for this recipe, but if you don't have one, you can just use any other kitchen appliance that can still juice the ingredients. Grate or finely chop the first 4 ingredients on the list or purchase freshly ground ones if they are available to make the juicing more convenient.

Ingredients:

2 cloves garlic
½ onion (small)
¼ teaspoon ground turmeric or 1 inch turmeric
¼ teaspoon ground ginger or ½ inch ginger
1 pc. lemon
½ jalapeño (small) or 1/16 teaspoon cayenne pepper
1 oz. apple cider vinegar
½ inch horseradish (optional)

Procedure:

Peel lemon and garlic, and put the first 6 ingredients into the juicer one by one. You may choose to add more jalapeño or cayenne and apple cider vinegar if you are able to handle more heat. Once you feel the symptoms of an infection, take 1 oz. of this tonic thrice a day. Prepare a glass of water just in case you need it.

Antibiotic Syrup

Ingredients:

3.5 oz. fresh lemon juice
1 clove garlic
2 tbsp. powdered ginger
2 tbsp. honey
½ tbsp. cinnamon
½ tbsp. ground chili peppers

Procedure:

Throw in and mix all the ingredients in a bowl except for the honey. Add the honey after mixing for 2-3 minutes. Let the syrup rest at room temperature for about 3 hours. Transfer it to an airtight glass container after and refrigerate. It is recommended to take 1 tbsp. of this syrup daily if you want to boost your immune system, but make sure you do so on an empty stomach. If you are sick, take 1 tbsp. thrice a day before your meals.

Thyme Cough Syrup

Bandages were medicated using thyme before modern antibiotics came about. Thyme was also used to treat respiratory infections by turning it into salve, tisane, syrup, tincture, or steam. If you are currently suffering from coughs, then you can skip your usual cough syrups and create your very own thyme cough syrup instead. If you want to get the best out of thyme, then you may even add a pinch of it to your morning tea to strengthen your immune system.

Aside from cough syrup, you may also use thyme as an additional ingredient for cookies. The recipe for it is provided in the next page, and though it may not directly fight illnesses at the point of need, it does make an excellent snack that will keep you healthy and free of infections.

Ingredients:

1 cup water
4 tablespoons thyme
1 teaspoon lemon juice
¼ cup honey

Procedure:

Boil the water and then pour it over the thyme. Let it sit for about 15 minutes and then strain. Add honey and lemon juice and refrigerate for up to one week and use as needed. It is recommended to drink 1-2 tablespoons of this syrup for adults and 1-2 teaspoons for children.

Lemon Thyme Cookies

Ingredients:

½ cup silvered almonds, blanched
2 tbsp. fresh lemon thyme leaves, with stems removed
½ tsp. salt
2 cups all-purpose flour, divided
1 cup unsalted butter
¼ cup powdered sugar
¼ cup granulated sugar
1 tsp. pure lemon extract
1 tsp. pure vanilla extract

Procedure:

Using a food processor or blender, create a nut-herb mixture by pulsing almonds, thyme, and 2 tbsp. flour for about 20 seconds until they look finely ground, but not pasty. Then, sift the remaining flour in a medium bowl and add in the salt. Put the nut-herb mixture into the bowl with sifted flour and set aside.

Cream sugar and butter for 2-3 minutes until light and fluffy. Then add the sifted flour mixture bit by bit until all the ingredients are well-combined. Finally, add the vanilla and lemon extracts. Chill the dough by rolling it out into a log about 2 inches in diameter and wrapping with plastic wrap. Place in the freezer for 2 hours before baking.

While waiting, pre-heat the oven to 300°F and line two cookie sheets with parchment paper. Take out the rolled cookie dough and cut into ¼-inch segments. Arrange them on the cookie sheet so that they are 1-inch apart. Place on the middle rack of the oven and bake for 30-35 minutes or until the edges are slightly brown. Remove from the pans and place on the cooling rack to cool before eating.

Honey Lemon Cough Syrup

Ingredients:

2 cups honey
1 pc. lemon

Procedure:

Pour 2 cups of honey into a saucepan and place over low heat until warm. Be careful not to boil as this could diminish the antibiotic properties of the honey. Meanwhile, in another saucepan, place the whole piece of lemon, cover with water and let boil for 2-3 minutes until the lemon is soft. Let the lemon cool until you can handle it and slice into smaller pieces. Add the lemon pieces to the honey and let cook over low heat for about an hour.

Finally, strain the lemon pieces from the mixture, making sure to remove all pieces especially the seeds. Let the mixture cool before storing in a bottle and keeping in the refrigerator. This cough syrup will store properly in the refrigerator for up to 2 months.

When needed, children should take half a teaspoon to one teaspoon of the cough syrup four times a day. Adults can take a dosage of as much as one tablespoon at least four times each day.

Lemon Thyme Chicken

Ingredients:

¼ cup olive oil
3 tbsp. garlic, minced
1/3 cup white wine
1 tbsp. lemon zest
2 tbsp. lemon juice
1 tsp. fresh thyme, minced
1 ½ tsp. dried oregano
4 pcs. chicken breast fillet
1 pc. lemon

Procedure:

Pre-heat your oven and prepare a 9-inch by 11-inch baking dish.

Place the olive oil in a saucepan and warm it over low heat. Add the minced garlic. Cook for about one minute while stirring. Make sure that the garlic does not turn brown. Turn the heat off then add the lemon zest, white wine, thyme, lemon juice and oregano. Mix together and pour over the baking dish.

Dry the chicken breasts using a paper towel. Put them on the baking dish over the oil mixture with the skin side up. Drizzle them using olive oil. Use salt and pepper as seasonings. Cut the remaining lemon into wedges and place in between the chicken pieces.

Finally, bake in the pre-heated oven for about 30-40 minutes. Cover the dish tightly with a piece of foil and let it rest for 10 minutes before serving.

Apple Spice Juice

Ingredients:

4 pcs. apples
1 pc. carrot
1 stalk celery
1 fresh dandelion root
½ pc. lemon
Pinch of cinnamon
Pinch of nutmeg

Procedure:

Remove the apple core and pass through a juicer along with the carrot, celery, and dandelion root. Add the juice of half a lemon, a pinch of cinnamon, and a pinch of nutmeg. Serve this juice immediately to enjoy.

Living Oil Flu Formula

Ingredients:

12 drops thieves essential oil blend
6 drops oregano essential oil
2 drops frankincense essential oil

Procedure:

Simply combine all ingredients and mix well before putting in a capsule. Make sure to use therapeutic grade essential oils to avoid any harmful effects. This recipe is very strong and is not recommended for the common colds or simple prevention, and should not be given to children below the age of 12. Adults are recommended to take one capsule every four hours at the onset of flu for three days. When the flu persists, continue taking the capsule once every eight hours for another four to six days.

Garlic and Onion Soup

Ingredients:

50 cloves organic garlic
2 tbsp. olive oil
2 tbsp. butter
2 pcs. red onion
1 tbsp. fresh thyme
6 cups chicken broth
3 cups stale bread, crushed
1 cup sour cream

Procedure:

Preheat your oven to 350°F. While waiting, prepare a baking dish that will hold your garlic pieces. Peel the garlic cloves and place them on the baking tray then drizzle with some olive oil and cover with foil. Place the dish in the pre-heated oven and cook for an hour and half. Let cool afterwards.

Heat the 2 tbsp. of olive oil and the 2 tbsp. of butter in a small saucepan over low heat. Peel the onion and dice before placing in the saucepan with the butter and oil. Let this cook for about 5 minutes with frequent stirring until the onion becomes soft and translucent.

Crush the cooked garlic and add to the saucepan with the onions. Mix well, then add the fresh thyme. Add in the crushed breadcrumbs and let cook for another 5 minutes before removing the thyme leaves and putting the mixture on the blender or food processor. Let the blender run until you have a smooth and creamy mixture then return to the saucepan and add a cup of sour cream. Season with salt and pepper and enjoy.

Shiitake Mushroom Soup

Ingredients:

8 cups vegetable broth
6 cups cauliflower, chopped
6 cups shiitake mushrooms, chopped
½ tsp. pink rock salt
1 tbsp. apple cider vinegar
2 cups onions, chopped

Procedure:

Combine all ingredients in a large pot and bring to a boil. Once boiling, lower the heat and let it simmer for 20 minutes. Finally, pass through the blender until you have a soup with smooth consistency. Enjoy this soup while warm and drizzle with some pesto for added flavor.

Sage Gargle Recipe

Ingredients:

2 tbsp. sage
2 cups boiling water
½ tsp. salt

Procedure:

Start by boiling 2 cups of water in a saucepan. Add the sage to the boiling water and let it steep for about 10 minutes. When finished, pour the liquid over a strainer to remove the herbs and stir in half a teaspoon of salt. Use this liquid as a gargle for sore throat and other infections.

Green Smoothie

Ingredients:

1 cup fresh parsley, including stem and leaves
¼ cup frozen pineapple
2 tsp. honey
1 inch ginger, peeled and grated
¼ cup plain yogurt
1 tbsp. lemon juice
¼ cup water

Procedure:

Combine all of the ingredients in a blender and add a few cubes of ice. Let the blender run until you have a smooth drink and transfer to a glass to enjoy. Drink this green smoothie to fight off respiratory infections and to help strengthen your immune system.

Antibiotic Juice

Fresh juices can easily save your life. Since these fruits and vegetables are in juice form, not only are they easy to consume, but the body will also absorb the nutrients easily. This recipe is recommended for those who are suffering from bronchitis, sinusitis, influenza, and other common infections because it is both an antibiotic and antiseptic. For best effects, drinking one glass daily is recommended.

Ingredients:

1 apple
1 beet
1 carrot
Pineapple slices (around 4 inch slices)
¼ inch ginger
¼ inch radish
1 pc. garlic
Procedure:

Wash all the ingredients. Cut each of them into very small pieces and then toss them into a blender or a juicer. Dilute the juice with half a glass of water before consuming.

Chapter 4 | Antiviral Recipes

Many people have to go through serious medication and even hospital confinement to have their viral infections treated. However, knowing a few antiviral recipes that you can make on your own can also prove to be effective and efficient. There are a number of natural remedies and recipes that anyone can try. However, before preparing these recipes, be sure to consult with an herbalist or have your herbal medicine guide ready. These recipes need to be precise in order for them to work properly and not go the wrong way. Also, every individual has his or her own specific needs so make sure to apply your own adjustments when necessary.

Cold and Flu Tonic

Ingredients:

1 part fresh garlic, chopped
1 part fresh onion, chopped
1 part fresh ginger root, grated
1 part fresh horseradish root, grated
1 part fresh cayenne peppers, chopped
Raw apple cider vinegar

Procedure:

Prepare your ingredients first by chopping the vegetables and grating the root crops. Also prepare your container, preferably a glass mason jar. Combine your ingredients and put them in the mason jar, filling it up to three-quarters of the way. Finally, top off with the raw apple cider vinegar until the jar is filled. Seal the lid and shake well to mix all the ingredients.

Set your tonic aside in a clean and dry place, making sure to shake it at least once a day for the next fourteen days. After the two weeks is over, filter your tonic by pouring it over a piece of clean cloth and transferring to another clean container. Make sure to label it properly and have it ready when the need arises. A recommended dosage of 1 to 2 ounces two times a day will help keep the infections away. If the infections are already present, increase your daily dosage to as much as 5 to 6 times a day. This tonic will last for years to come so go ahead and make your own today.

Onion Poultice

Ingredients:

2 pcs. organic onions
¼ cup organic ginger, grated
¼ cup filtered water

Procedure:

Peel and slice the onions and peel and grate ginger. In a saucepan, lightly sauté the onion and ginger in the filtered water. Cook only until the onions are soft and translucent, not browned. When done, pour over a strainer to remove the water then spread the onions and ginger in the middle of a dishtowel. Let it cool for a while or until it can be handled when placed on the skin.

To use the poultice, place it while warm on the chest to relieve congestion. You can also place the onion poultice at the bottom of the feet as an alternative. Leave it on for 20 minutes at a time. You can reheat the poultice for reusing purposes. You can expect coughing to occur shortly after the poultice is used as it expels the mucous from the lungs.

Antiviral Guacamole

Ingredients:

2 pcs. avocados, mashed
1 pc. medium tomato
½ pc. red bell pepper
1 pc. onion, minced
½ pc. small zucchini, grated
2 tsp. kelp
Pinch of salt

Procedure:

Prepare all the ingredients first by mashing the avocados, slicing the tomato into small pieces, chopping the red bell pepper finely, mincing the onion, and grating the zucchini. Combine all the chopped vegetables into a bowl, add the kelp, and then sprinkle with salt. Mix the ingredients properly and enjoy this antiviral guacamole with some crackers or by itself.

Lemon and Ginger Tea

Lemon is known as a detoxifying agent, but it also works extra time as a natural protection against infection. Having lemon in your drink or in your meal will help in cleansing your bowels and your liver, also helping to get rid of virus and bacteria.

Ingredients:

3 pcs. lemons
2 pcs. ginger nuggets (4 inches long each)
½ tablespoon cloves
3 pcs. cinnamon sticks
8 cups alkaline water
Coconut nectar (to taste)

Procedure:

Slice the lemons and ginger nuggets into thin pieces and place in a saucepan. Add the cloves to the pan, followed by the sticks of cinnamon, and finally cover with alkaline or spring water. Let the liquid simmer on low to medium heat for at least thirty minutes or until you see a yellow tint in the liquid. Once you see this color, your tea is ready. Pour into tea cups and enjoy with a teaspoon of coconut nectar to get a yummy and healing tea.

Antiviral Cocktail

Ingredients:

4-5 pcs. carrots
½ pc. organic cucumber
1 pc. garlic clove, with peel
1 pc. small turnip
1 cup watercress
1 pc. lemon, peeled

Procedure:

Prepare ingredients by washing them first. Remove the tops from the carrots, slice the cucumber into smaller pieces and peel the lemon. Let all ingredients pass through a juicer and enjoy immediately.

Elderberry and Cinnamon Syrup

Elderberry, also known as sambucus, is quite common in the subtropical regions around the world. Its abundance has perhaps led to its discovery as being an effective treatment against the influenza virus. Along with the flu, elderberry also works as a natural treatment for HIV virus and herpes simplex virus. The inherent property of the elderberry to fight off virus is also known to multiply through the cells, making it easier to recover and to stop the virus from spreading further throughout the body. Make your own natural remedy by following the recipe below and ward off viral diseases.

Ingredients:

2/3 cup black elderberries
3 ½ cups water
2 tablespoons fresh ginger root
1 teaspoon cinnamon powder
½ teaspoon cloves
1 cup raw honey

Procedure:

Combine the first five ingredients in a medium saucepan and bring to a boil. Remember not to put in the honey yet. Once the liquid has come to a boil, lower the heat and simmer for one hour. The liquid will have reduced to about half of its original volume. Let it cool until it can already be handled, then strain over a glass jar. Let the liquid cool to room temperature and finally add one cup of raw honey. Stir to combine and transfer to your preferred container. Stay protected from flu by taking one tablespoon of the syrup a day for adults and one teaspoon a day for kids. If you want to treat the flu, then take the dosage every 3 hours of the day until the flu symptoms disappear.

Immunity Soup

Ingredients:

1 ½ tsp. extra virgin olive oil
2 pcs. large onions
3 pcs. garlic cloves
1 tbsp. ginger
2 cups shiitake mushrooms
2 pcs. large carrots
2 ½ pcs. astragalus root
8 cups mushroom stock
2 tbsp. soy sauce
2 cups broccoli

Procedure:

Prepare ingredients by slicing the vegetables. Slice the onions into thin strips, smash the garlic and remove the peel, mince the ginger, slice the shiitake mushrooms thinly, slice the carrots into thin strips, and also slice the scallions into small pieces. Using a large pot, heat the olive oil over medium heat and add in the onions, ginger, and then the garlic. Sauté and cook for about 5 minutes. Throw in the mushrooms, the sliced carrots, and the astragalus root. Top off with 8 cups of stock and add another 2 cups of water. Turn on high heat and bring to a boil, then reduce to low heat and let simmer for 40 minutes.

Finish the soup by seasoning with the soy sauce and some salt, and then add in the broccoli and let simmer for another two minutes until the broccoli is cooked. Before serving, take out the astragalus roots.Antiviral Tonic

Ingredients:

1/8 cup garlic, chopped
1/8 cup onion, chopped
1/8 cup ginger, grated
1/8 cup horseradish, grated
1/8 cup hot peppers, chopped
Raw apple cider vinegar

Procedure:

Combine all ingredients except the apple cider vinegar in a clear jar, making sure that the jar is big enough only to be ¾ full once all the ingredients are in. When all the vegetables and peppers are in, fill the remaining ¼ space of the jar with apple cider vinegar. Seal tightly and shake well. Store the tonic in a cool and dry place for two weeks, making sure to shake it at least once every day. When the two weeks are over, strain over a clean piece of cloth and store in a bottle. Label properly.

Use the tonic by taking 1 to 2 ounces at least twice a day. For signs of infection, take the tonic five times a day.

Chicken Soup

Ingredients:

5 lbs. organic chicken for stewing
4 cloves garlic
10 carrots (large)
1 bunch parsley
3 parsnips
3 onions (large)
1 sweet potato (large)
2 turnips
6 stalks celery
1 tsp. celery seed
Hot pepper flakes
Salt and pepper to taste

Procedure:

Clean out the chicken and place in a large pot filled with 3 to 4 quarts of cold water. Bring to a boil and then add the garlic, carrots, parsley, parsnips, onions, sweet potato, turnips, and celery. Let the ingredients boil for approximately 1 and a half hour. Then, add the celery seeds and hot pepper flakes. Cook for 45 minutes. Remove the chicken from the soup. While you will not use the chicken any further for the soup, you may use it for stock at a later time. Add salt and pepper to taste.

Antiviral Tea

Ingredients:

4 cups water
1 tea bag Echinacea
1 sprig rosemary
2 tbsp. honey
3 tsp. elderberry syrup
2 cloves garlic, crushed or 2-3 drops wild oregano oil

Procedure:

Let water boil and then add the Echinacea tea bag and rosemary. Remove from heat and let the plant extracts infuse for about 2 to 3 minutes. When it has cooled, pass through a strainer and add the honey, elderberry syrup, and the garlic or oregano oil. Take this tea until the symptoms of infection disappear.

Homemade Healing Salve

If you are in search of homemade first aid recipes, then this homemade healing salve is for you. Not only does it smell heavenly, but it also works great on scrapes, burns and cuts.

Ingredients:

¼ cup coconut oil
¼ cup grapeseed oil
3 tbsp. beeswax pastillies
10 drops Melaleuca oil
8 drops lavender oil
5 drops vitamin E oil
5 drops lemon oil

Procedure:

Melt together the coconut oil, grapeseed oil, and beeswax at 350 °F for about 5 minutes. You may use a microwave or even an oven toaster to do so. Let it cool for a bit and then add in the Melaleuca oil, lavender oil, vitamin E oil, and lemon oil. Stir all the ingredients and transfer to a handy container.

Turmeric Smoothie

Ingredients:

1 cup coconut milk or hemp
1 banana
½ cup frozen mango or pineapple bits
1 tbsp. coconut oil
1 tsp. chia seeds
1 tsp. maca
½ tsp. turmeric
½ tsp. ginger
½ tsp. cinnamon

Procedure:

Toss in and mix all the ingredients in a blender until smooth. It is recommended to drink this smoothie daily before you eat your breakfast.

Conclusion

Thank you again for downloading this book!

I hope this book was able to help you better understand how antibiotics and antivirals work and how you can use various ingredients to create natural versions of them for treatment. While these recipes may take some time to prepare compared to just buying your usual prescription drugs, the long-term effects on your health certainly make them worth the extra effort. It's a good thing that you already know that you don't always have to rely on medications for the most common bacterial and viral infections.

Most of the ingredients mentioned here are probably already available in your home, so why don't you try making them? Besides, they are not only great in providing momentary relief to your illness, but they will also keep you strong and healthy in the long run.

Finally, if you enjoyed this book, please take the time to share your thoughts and post a review on Amazon. It'd be greatly appreciated!

Thank you and good luck!

I Need Your Help!

Please take a minute out of your busy schedule to leave a review.

Your review will let readers know what to expect and what you liked about this book. I am looking forward to reading your review.

Thank you so much for your feedback!

How to Submit a Review

To submit a review:

1. Make sure you are signed in.
2. Hover over **Your Account** in the upper right hand corner.
3. Click on **Your Orders**.
4. Click on **Digital Orders**.
5. Click **Write a customer review** in the Customer Reviews section.
6. Rate the item and write your review.
7. Click **Submit**.

How to submit a review from your Kindle device

Please follow the link below for instructions.

http://www.dummies.com/how-to/content/posting-an-amazon-book-review-from-your-kindle.html